Lessen the Stressin'

How to transform stress from a destructive enemy into a life enhancing ally.

By Charles F. Roost, D.C.

Acknowledgement:

I want to thank my wife, Judi for her input into this book, as well as into my life. She will, undoubtedly say that she had nothing to do with it. But she is the conduit for much of what God has taught me, and the example that raises me far above the person I would be without her.

She is a wonderfully sensitive and wise, godly person without whom I would be lost and confused. An encourager, a mirror, full of the Word and the Spirit of God.

Lessen the Stressin'

By Charles F. Roost, D.C.

Published in the United States of America by
  DC Publishing

ISBN **978-1515126898**

722 N. Creyts Rd.
Lansing, MI 48917
www.Delta-Chiro.com

Curriculum Vitae

Charles F. Roost, D.C.

1980   Palmer College of Chiropractic - Doctor of Chiropractic - Graduated Magna Cum Laude

1981- Present: Delta Chiropractic Center - Director/Owner - 35 years of practice – Over 1 million spinal adjustments

1984   American Disability Evaluation Research Institute, University of Michigan

1987-95   Fellow of the American Academy of Spinal Biomechanical Engineering

1989   Michigan Chiropractic Council - District II President

1990-91   M.C.C. State Board of Directors

1994-97   Christian Chiropractors Association – National Board of Directors

1995   CCA Chiropractor of the Year

1996-01   Chaplain - Christian Chiropractors Association

1990-95   Michigan Christian Chiropractors Assoc. - Founder and President

1984-05   National Association of Disability
Evaluating Physicians

1987-90   Scientific Advisory Board of AASBE

2007   Pro-Adjuster Certification Level III

2005-14   Global Outreach International –
Board Chairman

2011 – Present CCA Missions Committee
Chairperson

2014 - Present - Member of the Chiropractic
Advisory Board for Medical Professional Liability
Insurance Company

Author   -   Marianne

            -     Step Up To Better Health

            -     17 Questions

            -     The Rest of the Gospel

            -     Practicing Above the Treetops

            -     Lessen the Stressin'

Index

Key Points:

1) **Key Point #1:** Good stress prepares the mind and body for action

   a. Pg. 15

2) **Key Point #2:** What does stress do to us? It kills us.

   a. Pg. 30

3) **Key Point #3:** Stress causes physical and chemical changes – whether you notice them or not.

   a. Pg. 51

4) **Key Point #4:** Stress is everywhere! You cannot escape

   a. Pg. 68

5) **Key Point #5:** Life is charging, and charging downhill.

   a. Pg. 77

6) **Key point #6:** Less stress means better health.

   a. Pg. 109

7) **Key Point # 7:** There are specific, practical ways to deal with the chemical soup.

    a. Pg. 120

8) **Key thought #8:** There are real and practical benefits to lowering our stress level.

    a. Pg. 125

9) **Key Point #9:** There is actually a "sweet spot" of stress level that allows us maximum effectiveness in life.

    a. Pg. 129

Introduction:

Stress is an odd thing; universally blamed for everything from broken relationships to lost productivity, to most every illness and disease known to man. But we all know that stress is bad. We all know that it causes serious health issues. We all know that it's just about everywhere. But we all seem to think we don't really have it.

One way to make the impact of stress real to us is to ask some important questions about stress:

1) What is stress?
2) How does it do that?
3) What causes my stress?
4) What does stress do to my health?
5) Is it possible to get rid of or lower stress?
6) How do I manage the stress that I'm stuck with?
7) What are the benefits to lowering stress?

8) Are there any hidden costs of lowering or managing stress?

We are going to answer these questions in practical detail. Together, we are going to come to the realization that stress is manageable, and that it can be transformed from a destructive enemy into a life enhancing ally. We are going to take stress out of the "We all know that..." realm, which is so impersonal and distant, and into the practical and personal, "Ah, now I know how to..." moment.

Chapter 1 – Stress – Our Friend

I saw a patient this week who was under such pressure from family issues she could not sleep, she was experiencing chest pains, she was unable to eat, interact with people, or even make plans for the day. The stress was literally killing her.

The next day, I met with a man who had a similar family situation, siblings fighting and threatening lawsuits over inheritance issues. This guy slept fine at night, made plans for the situations that were arising with his family, and enjoyed time with his immediate family each evening.

What is the difference? Do we have a choice in how we will respond to stress? Or is it written in our genes, hardwired into our nerves to either stress out, or chill out?

The exact same stress may impact two people entirely differently. So what is the deal with stress? Where does stress get the authority to rule and ruin one life, and yet remain safely contained within reasonable boundaries in another?

Stress is good and bad

Scenario One:

Feeling the stress of the upcoming presentation, Fred was compelled to push through the tedious monotony of the warm afternoon, and run through his power point one more time. As he walked into the board room, the afternoon sun slanting through the vertical blinds looked to him like arrows pointing toward the white board on which he would soon diagram his future. Alert, and ready, he stepped through his jitters, stood tall, and began sharing his vision for the next phase of company growth.

Scenario Two:

As the man in the watch cap emerged from the shadows of the alley, Kate felt the impact of adrenaline dumping into her blood stream. Her muscles tightened, her breathing grew more shallow and quick. She tightened her grip on her purse and walked with quicker steps past the dark opening to the right of the sidewalk. The man quickened his pace to close with her, but as he reached out to grab her shoulder, Kate spun on her toes, batted his arm to the side, and kicked him in the groin, just as she had imagined she should in such an instance. The man grunted, his knees buckled, and Kate spun again and ran for the safety of the coffee shop at the end of the block.

These two scenarios demonstrate what stress can do for us when confronted with situations that push us outside of our normal routines. These situations illustrate what could be called "good stress", not because the circumstances were good, but because the body's reaction to the stressors helped Fred and Kate to respond to the situation in a positive, productive way.

Key Point #1: Good stress prepares our mind and body for action.

When faced with a challenge, stress gives us what we need to face and overcome challenges that push us outside our normal experience. As we will see in the next chapter, stressors in our environment, or in our experiences, or even in our minds, cause glands and tissues to release chemicals that are essential and healthy – in the right scenarios, but dangerous and damaging when proper outlet is not available.

So let's look at another facet of the stress response.

Scenario Three:

Feeling the stress of the upcoming presentation, Frank was compelled to push through the afternoon, fighting the exhaustion, and grinding through his power point one more time. As he walked into the board room, the afternoon sun slanting through the vertical blinds jabbed at his eyes like arrows pointing toward the white board on which his career hung. Tense and weary at the same time, he felt the sweat bead his forehead. He walked toward the front of the room, feeling the tension in his muscles, and the pressure building in his head and chest. His tongue glued to his mouth as he searched for words to begin.

Scenario Four:

As the man in the watch cap approached from the shadows of the alley, Kitty felt the impact of adrenaline dumping into her blood stream. Her muscles tightened, her breathing grew more shallow and quick. She tightened her grip on her purse and walked with staccato steps past the dark opening to the right of the sidewalk. The man quickened his pace to close with her, and as he reached out to grab her shoulder, Kate screamed. Paralyzed by her fear, she felt her knees buckle, and she crumpled to the cement, just as she had imagined she would in such an instance. The man laughed as he tore her purse from her numb fingers. Kitty stared helplessly at the safety of the coffee shop at the end of the block.

Hm. The same scenarios – completely different outcomes. The same stimuli produced the very same chemicals, injecting them into the blood stream of Fred and Frank, and Kate and Kitty in microseconds. Yet those chemicals contributed to very different outcomes.

Didn't we already know that?

We will see, in coming chapters, how stressors will bring out the 'better' in us, or the 'break point' in us. The outcome of that chemical response all depends on . . . Read on to find out.

Chapter 2: What Stress Does To Us

Scenario Five:

As the condition of Joseph's son worsened, he found it more and more difficult to concentrate. Joseph began to find it hard to make good decisions – or any decision at all, for that matter. The stress grew stronger as his son's situation grew worse. Drained of energy, buried in apathy, his business failed, compounding the stress even further.

So, while stress can be our friend, it can just as easily become an enemy. At the onset of a stressful experience, certain powerful chemicals will be dumped into the blood stream, but depending on genetics, life style, and attitude, those chemicals will result in different outcomes, such as:

- High blood pressure, leading to a devastating cerebro-vascular incident
- Pre-game jitters, bringing out the highest level of competition
- Mental acuity that keeps us sharp before we present or perform
- Acid-etching of the stomach, resulting in a medium ripe for ulcers

The graph below depicts the fact that stress takes a toll.

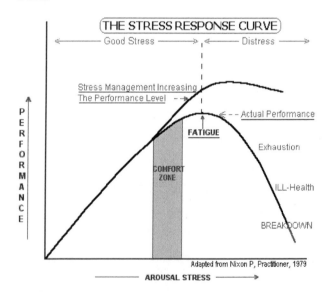

Adapted from Nixon P, Practitioner, 1979

Let's talk about how the monster called stress causes such mayhem.

In the next chapter we'll see that there is a "sweet spot" amount of stress that brings out the good without triggering the bad. But there is also a way to learn to respond to stressors that will tilt the odds in favor of using stress to our advantage.

For now, understand that stressors, good or bad, directly trigger glandular activity in our bodies that release strong chemicals into our blood stream that enable higher level of function, and prepare the rest of our organs for increased activity.

Muscles will contract more quickly, the heart will pump more blood, the brain synapses will come up to a higher level of acuity, and the digestive system slows down to save resources for what's needed right at that moment. In fact, the glandular response to stressors is quick – very quick. Within one hundredth of a second, the chemistry throughout the entire body changes, and you've felt it happen.

Think back to a recent example of your own. Recall a time when you were suddenly frightened, or embarrassed, or confronted. Think about how quickly you felt your face flush, your body warm, you started sweating, and your chest tightened. It is amazing how fast the chemicals are released, dumped into the body, and circulated to impact the function of your whole body.

I experienced this recently when, for reasons that are complicated, I had to go through a polygraph examination. During this examination, the examiner asked a question that triggered a memory which, in turn, triggered a stress response, and within less than a second, I felt my body go into hyper-stress mode. I felt my breathing quicken, my face flush, my hands sweat, my chest tighten. The examiner asked, "What was *that* all about?" He knew right away, from the readings on his computer, that I had experienced an intense stress response.

This happens so quickly because the glands that secrete these chemicals are prepared beforehand.

They produce the chemicals in small amounts while you are at ease, and store them against the moment when needed. Then, at the right trigger, the glands contract, injecting the chemicals directly into the blood stream where they circulate immediately throughout the body. Blood scoots along your arteries, capillaries and veins, speeding through your entire body every minute or so, achieving speeds of up to 10 mph. So, to get from your adrenal glands to your brain, a distance of about three feet – adrenalin gets there in about a second. From your adrenals to your heart, it takes only a small fraction of that.

The stress chemicals are used for what is called the "Fight or Flight" response. This is named such, because they prepare your body to respond in one of those two ways. We are suddenly hyped up and ready to either physically fight back against an attacking enemy, or to turn tail and skedaddle away, running to save our skin.

This is all as planned. It is a normal and healthy event. Those chemicals and hormones are crucial for our best response to the situation at hand. While this is obvious in situations that require a physical response, they are useful for mental response analogous to fighting back or running away, also. In our modern, protected society, we are less likely to have to defend ourselves from a hunting lion than we are a hunting lawyer. We are less likely to have to run away from an attacking Hun warrior than we are to have to run from a persistent bill collector. Physical fighting and escaping are much less common in our modern, urban jungles. But the chemical / stress response is the same, and knowing what to do about it is crucial to our wellbeing.

So, the chemical soup sloshes around our arteries, veins, and interstitial fluid, bathing the cells and organs. The chemicals never get burned up in battle, never used up to fuel a sprint to safety, but continue circulating in a toxic sludge that causes gradual, but serious and dangerous changes in our physiology and health. The chemicals are designed to spur our tissues into action, and they will have their effect. But if the action spurred is not significant physical activity, it will be something else – something as significant as fighting, but more subtle. Something as health-impacting as running for your life, but more insidious. Something as deadly as staying alive in a dangerous situation, but more gradual.

Yes, those chemicals must be used up, or they persist there, circulating in a chemical soup in our blood stream. And if they stay there, unused for the purpose for which they were called forth, they will be used in other, damaging ways.

So what are these chemicals? What is in the cocktail of hormones that gives us the life-saving, or damaging stress response? What is produced by the adrenal, hypothalamus, thyroid and other glands that can be so important to our survival in a dangerous situation, yet so dangerous in a gentler setting?

Stressors, experienced by our mind or body, are noted by the brain, which instantly sends messages to the adrenal glands, saying, "Danger! Danger! Give us some juice!" And the adrenal glands instantly respond by squeezing out the chemicals that supercharge our muscles, heart and brain into hyper action status.

Adrenalin comes from the adrenal glands, Thyroxin from the Thyroid gland, Cortisol and other Corticosteroids, Testosterone, and hundreds (some sources say over 1,800 different chemicals!) of other subtle chemicals are produced by other tissues. And all of themheighten the body's ability to burn energy in a way that will improve the odds of surviving a dangerous encounter.

Within microseconds, these supercharged chemicals are injected into the bloodstream, and are immediately circulated to:

- the heart, where they stimulate stronger contractions,

- the muscles, where they encourage blood flow and stronger contractile availability,

- the stomach and intestines, where they slow digestive processes, freeing blood and nutrients and oxygen to go where they are more immediately needed,

- the brain, where they increase blood flow to the hind-brain, encouraging synapses to fire in ways that benefit the survival skills of fighting and running,

- the walls of the blood vessels themselves where they increase blood flow in peripheral muscles, and constrict blood flow in digestive and reproductive organs, and

- all of the cells where they alter energy manufacturing processes in the mitochondria to produce short term bursts of energy necessary for all of the functions above.

And this is all good! If we are to run from a tiger, or fight an attacking enemy, we need all of the above in order to raise our chances of coming out alive.

But, if we are getting all of this 'move juice' in response to a law suit, or a bill collector, or a lost job, those chemicals don't get used up. They simply continue to circulate around and around in our blood vessels looking for a place to energize. They continue to soak our cells in the chemical soup that turns toxic and drives extremely negative and dangerous physiological changes such as fat deposition around organs, lipid deposits inside blood vessels, and systemic inflammation.

These terms, fat deposition, lipid deposits, and inflammation sound distant and clinical, yet they are the harbingers of dramatic and life threatening processes. They are the 'four horsemen' of chronic diseases that we learn about when we hear statistics on the great killers of our culture: heart disease, stroke, and cancer. They are the drivers of the run-away train of inflammation in arthritis, and other systemic "algia"s like fibro-myalgia, and rheumatoid arthritis. And they are the mill stones around the neck of our immune systems, dragging down to ineffectiveness our ability to fight infectious invaders off, from simple colds to meningitis to cancer.

The implications to individual health, simply from stress, are huge. The implications to our society are catastrophic. It is estimated that well over 80% of doctor visits are driven by stress related illness. 80% of all doctor visits!

According to **lesstress.net**,

> Stress is very expensive and dangerous. Just glance through these stress facts:
>
> - It is estimated that American businesses lose approximately $200-$300 billion dollars per year to stress related productivity loss and the treatment costs of stress-related illnesses.
>
> - Every week, 95 million Americans suffer some kind of stress

related symptoms for which they take medication.

- A 20-year study conducted by the University of London concluded that unmanaged reactions to stress were a more dangerous risk factor for cancer and heart disease than either cigarette smoking or high cholesterol foods."

- Cost in percent of GDP

- Cost to US industry of stress-related illness is over $200 billion a year

- Each individual in the USA spends an average of $8,600 each year on health care.

- 17.1% of our GDP is spent on health care.

Key Point #2: What does stress do to us? It kills us.

Slowly or quickly – through cancer or stroke, it kills us.

It costs us – through inability to function or debilitating disease, it costs us.

But we already knew that, didn't we?

Knowing it is true is important. But it's not enough. It must stop. And it can stop. Let's look at how it causes all of this damage, then we'll look at how to stop it.

Chapter 3: The Mechanism of Stress Damage

Scenario Six: Martha tried to eat as healthy as she could. She stayed away from too much sugar. She avoided fats. She never drank more than one soda a day. And she had lots of fruits and veggies every day. Yet she weiged 192 pounds, and her blood sugar and cholesterol were out of control Her weight was carried in her hips and abdomen, and she could not lose the pounds or the inches, no matter how she starved herself.

Stress can be very obvious, intense, and it can feel – well – stressful. But stress is usually rather subtle and unobtrusive until it becomes an acute issue demanding our attention NOW! But even in the subtle stages, stress impacts our lives in predictable ways. And the specific mechanisms for stress impacting our health are well documented. This mechanism has been researched and documented and named – the General Adaptative

Syndrome. (Unfortunately the acronym for this life-changing issue is G.A.S. undermining the seriousness of the issue.) We will elect to avoid using that acronym here, so just get used to the wordy title.

General Adaptative Syndrome occurs in three stages if the system is working properly.

Stage One: Stress Alarm Reaction : *The initial effects of stress on the body.*

This is more commonly known as the '*fight or flight*' response. As soon as our body is faced with a stressful situation, our body explodes with a sudden surge of energy by intentionally flooding hundreds of hormones and chemical activators into the blood stream. We become alert and ready to meet any threat.

The main receptors of this chemical super-charge at this stage are heart, lungs, brain, nervous system and the muscles, all stimulated by this release of hormones. This system-wide arousal is initiated by the hypothalamus gland in the release of endorphins, the natural painkillers. At the same time, adrenaline is secreted by the adrenal glands. Adrenaline causes raised heart rate, increased blood pressure and the release of vital nutrients. It also causes muscle readiness, in the form of tension, and causes breathing to accelerate faster, yet grow shallower.

Nor-adrenaline is also secreted, and is associated with positive excitement. Another hormone, Cortisol, converts glycogen stored in the liver into blood sugar, thus stimulating the brain and whole body with instant energy.

In males, the hormone Testosterone is released, and provides a surge of raw strength. Thyroxin, released by thyroid gland, stimulates the metabolic system and regulates the oxygen consumption. Our digestive system slows down, as blood is diverted to essential organs required to meet the immediate threat. Thus the stress alarm reaction puts the body in the fight or flight mode.

In moments, depending on whether the stressor continues to trigger this response, the body shifts to the next level of reaction to stress.

2. Stage Two Of Stress Resistance: *The internal response to stress*

Once the alarm reaction is established and the immediate threat is over, the body moves into a stress resistance phase, where the bodily functions that were put on high-alert are reverted back to a near normal state. The heart rate, respiratory rate and metabolic activities come down to a maintenance level; but body is still ready and alert.

More cortisol, thyroxin etc are released to speed up the tissue repair systems, to address any body parts which may have been damaged during the encounter with the stressor. This is the stage of Stress Resistance, and while the immediate threat from the environment is over, the body is still going through a clear and predictable pattern of response to the stressor that started the process.

3. Stage Three: Stress Exhaustion : *Stress effect on the body turns harmful.*

This is the post-stress collapse. It is commonly referred to by the saying, "What doesn't kill you makes you stronger." It can be sudden, producing a shock-like weakness, or it may be gradual and greatly prolonged, resulting in chronic weariness and lack of energy.

Even without external threats, emotions such as anger, anxiety, fear and impatience are continuous stress stimulators, and without our knowledge, our body is put in (and stays in!) the 'fight or flight' mode. Overdose, or chronic levels of adrenaline often cause additional irritability and uneasiness. On top of that, a chronic production of nor-adrenaline makes us feel disconnected and high.

Too much of cortisol will suppress the immune system, making us vulnerable to a host of diseases. Extra sodium is retained, affecting the cardiovascular and excretory systems adversely.

Thus our body goes into stress exhaustion and tissue breakdown from the side effects of continuous, uncontrolled stress chemicals circulating in the blood system, seeping into the fluids between the cells (interstitial fluids), and invading and impacting the cells themselves. When this continues over days, weeks and months, emotionally, we become depressed, anxious, disoriented, insecure and frustrated. If this situation is allowed to proceed unchecked, we will see how family breakdown, mental illness, work absence, alcoholism or drug dependency can gradually encompass a life to further complicate the stress condition.

These stages occur on their own, though the intensity may vary depending upon our coping capabilities.

Psychologists say we respond to stress at two major levels: Consciously and Subconsciously.

1. Subconscious, "primary" evaluation of the threat:

At this level, we quickly:

- Decide if the situation is threatening – though this happens consciously at times, it takes place subconsciously in most situations. It is critical to respond too quickly to trust the slow-motion conscious processes to deal with the threat.

- Instantly evaluate our internal and external resources to deal with the problem – again, this happens within split seconds, and is done subconsciously.

- And without conscious awareness, choose what to do – this may happen as a reflex, without thinking it through, but the forebrain does have the opportunity to weigh in on the decision before we commit to reflex actions such as swinging a fist, or running.

So, much of this process happens subconsciously. And the ramifications are huge as they impact our long-term health. Thus we must do something to limit the impact of the stress, and to deal with the aftermath of the subconscious decisions we just made.

2. Conscious "secondary" evaluation:

Only now do we take the time to consciously, using our awareness and logical thinking processes:

• Evaluate of our efforts to deal with the stressful situation: has it worked this time? How about in the past?

• Continue to appraise the situation, reevaluating our primary response, until the threat is no longer present or felt.

• Act to clean up the results of our actions. For instance, if we were injured in the attack (the stressor event), we will now need to get care for the damage.

This level of response is slower and more consciously undertaken. We think through what we are doing, how we are responding, and if it is a beneficial response or not. We are likely to feel less stress if we feel competent to deal with any given situation. We are likely to feel more stress if we feel the event has taken us into circumstances we are not trained to handle. For example, if our supervisor gave us a project that was beyond our skill set, and thus caused stress, what can we do now to change that situation? Other factors, such as illness, exhaustion, addictions, and other lifestyle habits that we use to insulate our conscious mind from the subconscious, can also increase our stress over situations that we might otherwise take in a stride.

All along, during this process, our body, with all of its complicated physiology, responds in myriads of ways. And the impact of this chemical blitz has far-reaching consequences, some of which are obvious, and others of which are subtle and time-delayed but no less important.

Interestingly, there are normal wave patterns in hormones, including all the hormones that impact our sleep cycles, our moods, our relationships, our romance, our appetite and metabolism, and more. These normal daily variations vary with the time of day, the amount of light we are bathed in, noise levels, vibrations, our posture, our words, our choice of thoughts, and usually vary gradually as the patterns and activities of our daily lives change.

However, when stress hits us, this delicate dance of hormone balance can change in abnormal ways, at abnormal speeds, causing abnormal physiological balances. The dump of these chemicals can occur in as little as $1/100^{th}$ of a second, and those chemicals can speed through the body along the blood highways in seconds.

We've already seen that these chemical changes impact our bodies in huge ways. And if the chemicals are not used up through exercise or other stress management techniques, they will cause longer term issues.

If these acute episodes of stress response continue, they turn into chronic stressors, bringing a whole host of further chronic stress issues. Let's dig into some of these concerns next.

The normal cycles of hormone and chemistry changes can be mapped out over time. These waves look smooth and calm. They are relatively regular, and are predictable based on the factors of time of day listed above.

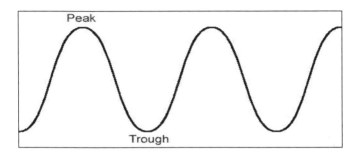

However, under times of stress, some of the waves turn into sharp, even jagged waves that even look damaging on their graphed form. In fact, the hormone levels represented by the waves are indeed damaging if left unmanaged.

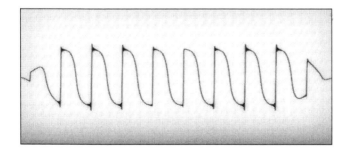

Health issues that occur at this stage of stress can include immediate symptoms and responses such as:

- Increased, shallow breathing
- Tightening of muscles, including tightening of abdominal muscles, tense arms and legs,
- Clenched jaw causing gritting of teeth.
- Sweating
- Dyspepsia
- Increased frequency of urine
- Irritability
- Back pain
- Anxiety
- Constipation or diarrhea
- Abnormal stomach acid levels
- Poor sleep
- Fatigue
- Headaches
- Loss of appetite
- Weight gain (ironically, considering the previous mentioned loss of appetite)

These "Primary" physical issues are irritating and impact our lives in fairly small ways. But it gets worse. If the stress continues, either from repeated acute sources such as repeated shocks or traumas, or from long term, unchanging stresses such as difficult work situations or chronic financial circumstances, the adrenal gland just keeps pumping out cortisol until the gland "burns out" and the waves flatten out. Non responsive. No resources remaining.

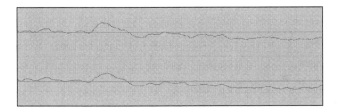

Of course, when this happens, the body has lost one of its main modes of compensating for stress, and this will lead to very difficult health issues, indeed.

From this point, the body has very little control, or regulation, over the production of the stress chemicals. A tipping point has been reached beyond which there is a cascade of issues, focusing on the unique weak links in each individual's physiology. Stress finds the weak link, the chink in the 'health armor' of each person, and brings that weak system, and the attendant symptoms to the surface. So for one it may cause ulcers, in another, high blood pressure, in another intractable headaches.

Following are some of the physical effects of stress on our body. They are all caused by the impact of the stress hormones, circulating at abnormally high levels, for sustained amounts of time, in our blood stream. Remember, the chemical soup is toxic, and can cause many negative physiological results in the body. There are three layers of impact from the stress chemicals when they are left circulating in the blood stream.

The first, or Primary responses were listed above. Secondary results from chronic stress include:

- Visceral fat deposition
- Palpitation : increased heart beat
- Tremors
- Cold, clammy extremities
- Constipation
- Diarrhea
- Hyperacidity
- Weakness
- Hair loss
- Lower thyroid hormones
- Lower immunoglobulin levels
- Hormone imbalances
- Testosterone, estrogen, insulin, etc.
- Neurotransmitters
- Moods, tension, depression, memory
- Low bone density
- Blood sugar imbalances
- High oxidative stress – rust in the cells
- Chronic inflamation

- High cholesterol

- Depression

- High blood pressure

- Insomnia

- Shortness of breath

- Stiff neck

- Upset stomach

- Ulcers

- Weight gain or loss

- Cancer

- Compromised Immune system

- Sleep stress - apnea

Finally, these already-significant health issues result in a third, or "Tertieary" level of health, social, and cultural problems. These "tertiary results" are devastating on an individual basis, and just as much so when multiplied by the thousands across a society.

Tertiary Results Of Chronic Stress:

- Self Medication – people who get no relief seek to cover the symptoms with behaviors which become addictive over time. Alcohol, street drugs, and behavioral addictions such as gambling bring numbing and relief for the short term.
- Substance abuse
- Over Medication – prescription meds can also come to be abused in a desperate effort to find relief.
- Problems with relationships
- Frequent Illnesses – compromised immunities leave sufferers susceptible to repeated, chronic, and progressive infectious diseases.
- Loss of effectiveness, concentration, and poor decision making, lead to loss of work and unemployment, and the attendant drift toward poverty
- Higher expenses and debt – the most common cause of personal bankruptcy is debt incurred from seeking health care.
- Generational Trends of poverty, abuse, etc.

We have listed a number of responses that occur as a result of the chemical soup. Note that some of those changes are temporary, and some are permanent.

Temporary changes will transition as the chemistry courses through our blood stream. Heart rate, digestive changes, blood pressure spikes, and soaring energy resources will quickly reach a peak in strength, and then fall back to normal levels as the chemicals disburse through our cells.

Over time, the permanent changes build and build, as fat is deposited around inner organs, cholesterol is layered along our arteries, and calcium is leached from our bones. These gradual changes are slow to reverse, so we consider them permanent. They can be undone, but it will take months or even years of work at reversing the impact of months and years of chronic stress and its corresponding cortisol abuse.

Key Point #3: Stress causes physical and chemical changes – whether you notice them or not.

But, hey, we already knew that.

Chapter 4: Causes of Stress

It is obvious that stress is ubiquitous. Without fail, when I ask a group if they have enough stress, they always chuckle, roll their eyes, groan. And when I offer to share mine if they feel they don't have enough, I have yet to get a taker for the deal.

Some, however, respond to my question by saying that they have no stress. But what they really mean is that they don't feel stressed. But as they tell me about their life, it is obvious that they have stress, sometimes a lot of it, even though they don't feel stressed out. They are still thinking that stress is the feeling of tension, rather than the real definition of stress, which is "The chemical response within the body to any external or internal stressor."

There are many causes of stress. For the sake of simplicity, let's look at physical, and then emotional sources of stress.

The most obvious causes of stress may be physical events that shock or 'stretch' or – well – stress the body. Physical causes of stress are mainly due to life style, environmental factors, or willing choices of activities undertaken.

Stress occurs when the demands upon an individual surpass the resources in their ability to live under such demands.

A. Life Style Stress:

- *Sedentary life style:* If the majority of your day is either sitting, lounging, or standing in one place, you have a lifestyle stress source. Lack of motion is subtle, and addictive, and will predispose you to many diseases like obesity, diabetes, increased cholesterol (with all of its dangers), and more. Toxins from body metabolism are produced in the body. These toxins accumulate, particularly in fat cells, and these toxins poison cells, organs and entire systems. I say the lifestyle is addictive, because it is progressive, it is harder and harder to change once it settles in, and it is resistant to any changes even when we recognize the damage it is doing.

- *Fast foods:* In our culture we have a very real addiction to fast foods. For instance, I can find at least 20 fast food outlets within a five minute drive from my office. Fast foods are full of artificial colors, flavors, fillers and simple carbohydrates. Each of these ingredients take more out of the body's reservoir of resources than they replace, sapping the system of important nutrients that could have been used to rebuild healthy tissues.

- *Fast Lives:* Go. Go! GO! This is the mantra of many a stressed life. Our culture subtly frowns on down time. Time spent just "being" is wasted when that same time could be invested in "doing". We've all heard the saying that we are not "human doings", but human beings. Yet we resent quiet time in everyone – except our kids during their nap time.

B. Environmental exposure to chemical stressors in fertilizers, pesticides, insecticides, and additives, as well as use of drugs (prescription, OTC, and street drugs), poison the system. And all of them have side effects, not to mention drug-drug interactions, are frequent and significant causes of stress in our lives. Radiation, toxic wastes, chemicals, impure air, and poor water sources add to the stress burden. On top of that is the big unknown: what will genetically modified foods do to our health? We are experimenting with the greatest petri dish in history as we introduce these new genes into the population across the entire globe. I get stressed just thinking about it.

C. A 'Driven' Lifestyle is a mindset of 'never enough'. This sense that our motor is constantly revving, that we must do more, accomplish more, and accumulate more than our neighbor will never be satisfied. Giving in to it will drive our stress level through the roof. This mindset is called workaholism, and it can often be found in a career, but just as easily in volunteering, and often is the result of needing to hide from inner pain by being busy. This hurtful habit depletes our bodies' reserves and leads to exhaustion, susceptibility to disease and more of the effects noted in the last chapter.

Excessive exercise is another aspect of a driven lifestyle that can cause stress. While exercise can be used to help manage stress, taken to a higher level of compulsion, stress becomes a stressor in its own right. Pounding the pavement, and your joints, hour after hour, obsessing over getting to the gym every day (or twice a day), obsessing on getting heart rate, or BMI, or fat ratio to the next level, or making sure the scale doesn't tip past that next digit – these are indicators that we may have allowed exercise to drive us, rather than using exercise to maintain health.

D. Poor Attention to Health Habits: Because of our driven lives, we often forget the essential requisites of refilling our health reservoir with positive input. Purposefully filling our lives with positives such as fresh air, pure water, regular exercise, and sun exposure is crucial to cleansing our lives of stress.

Further, drinking half your body weight in ounces of water every day is essential for absorption of nutrients, metabolism, and removal of toxins.

E. Chronic Illness is another source of stress in an individual. Suffering through day after endless day, pain, lack of progress, lack of sleep, and loss of hope all contribute to stress, which in turn detract from the body's ability to heal. Just as importantly, illness in loved ones also produces stress and anxiety in an individual.

F. Financial Stress: Debt is highly stressful for any individual. And once begun, the trend toward more and more debt is hard to stop, much less correct. Inflation, insufficient income, lack of other sources of income, ineffective saving habits, habitual spending, and failure in business all contribute to the quagmire of debt. Like tar, sticking to your fingers, once you touch it, debt and financial stress spreads its dark smear all around.

G. Trauma: An accident that causes our body to react to an acute or significant amount of physical damage is a source of stress in several ways. Not only the damage and pain, themselves, but the interruption of our schedule, the added financial burden, and the trauma itself, all trigger the same chemical issues that other stressors do.

H. Vibration and noise: Our modern culture is so full of vibration and noise that we don't even recognize it anymore. I went on a hike in the far north of Michigan. Alone on a trail, I stopped for a moment and gradually realized that I was feeling nervous. As I stood alone in that moment, I finally realized that it was absolutely silent. A feeling that I had not experienced in years. Absolutely no sound penetrated the deep woods that I found myself in. No cars, no aircraft, no train, no hum of air conditioner or heater. No voices, no radio or T.V., no barking dog, and no buzz of a computer tower at my feet. As we travel, by car, bus or airplane, there are constant vibrations, subtle and finely balanced, that keep our body in constant alert status without our ever recognizing it. These vibrations, and the background noises of modern life keep whispering in our ears, "Go. Go. Go."

I. Inactivity: Ironically, inactivity can also be a physical stressor. If we sit too long, our bodies respond in ways similar to the reactions triggered with a driven lifestyle. Apparently there is a balance between too busy, and bored.

J. Toxins: Tobacco, alcohol, sugar, caffeine, immunizations, fluorine, and more, our culture is bathed in chemistry that is toxic to our systems. Some still argue that there are good reasons for some of these chemical that we willingly take into our bodies, but nobody can convince me that there is a minimally acceptable level of mercury, arsenic, tar, or even fluorine that we should willingly ingest. And while we tolerate these toxins up to a point, each exposure to yet another toxin is an onslaught on our systems' ability to decontaminate and rise above the mess in which we live.

Emotional sources of stress are just as impactful as physical ones. What happens in the mind is just as real as an actual physical occurrence. Our body reacts the same way to a clearly imagined situation as it does to a physical situation. In fact, it has been said that an imagined event is completely indistinguishable to the mind from a 'real' event, if that imagined event is pictured in enough detail. This is helpful when doing proactive activities such as goal setting, but damaging and harmful when referring to stressful emotional events.

Inner wounds that we carry around, difficult family relationships, a verbally abusive boss, a co-worker who you wish you could hide from, things that happen to us that shouldn't, or things that should have been poured into our lives, but weren't – such as a lack of nurture, lack of love, lack of support or security.

Following is a list of examples of **emotional** stressors that impact our lives with the same chemical results as physical stresses.

A. Daily Incidental Stress: Driving to and from the workplace everyday is an additional stress all by itself, and can contribute to the daily load of stress that an individual has to carry about. And with tight schedules, packed calendars and too much to do, a flat tire, a locked car, a friend needing help, or a sudden illness can push the schedule beyond its flex point in a moment.

Traffic delays, lost keys, abusive fellow drivers, a fender bender, and parking tickets are still more examples of incidental stressors that add to the problem, and the body responds with a new dose of the chemical toxins, just as it does with physical stressors.

B. Difficult Relationships are even more stressful, because they don't disappear when we walk away for a few hours. Our minds continue to stew over the challenges, slowly producing the 'wonder-drugs' cortisol and its cohorts, adding to and strengthening the chemical stew.

C. Time Pressure: Our culture is insistent in its demands to do more, produce more, to go and go some more. This pressure, and the nearly complete lack of down time is another example of a lifestyle that presses our minds into the mode of stress. Part of this is our fault, shown in the difficulty of saying the simple word, 'no'. We load one event on top of another, one more responsibility on top of an already-full schedule, and our adrenal glands try to help by doing their job – churning out more cortisol to keep us going.

Many of the events we take on are voluntary and good, charitable activities. Some are laid on us by the demands of work or family. But in either case there are limits. At some point we overload and step into the stressful zone of too much.

D. Multi-tasking: Due to the issues of too much to do, with too little time to do it, we often answer the 'siren call' of multi-tasking. We decide that if we can accomplish two tasks at the same time, we can lighten the load. For instance, why not play with my toddler, while talking to my mother, and downloading the pictures from our vacation?

Well, two things occur when we do more than one task at a time. First, we lose efficiency. The brain is only capable of thinking about one thing at a time, so while we think we are doing several things at once, we are really only switching from one task to the next, over and over. And with each 'switch' between simultaneous tasks we lose 40% of our productivity with each task. And, while we may not need 100% of our mental capacity to do any of the individual tasks, the toll adds up when we end up using only 60% or less on each one. We fool ourselves into thinking that we are doing our best, but each task suffers. The toddler gets subtle clues that they are not really important, mom ends the call feeling that something is 'off', and the pictures get misfiled, or accidentally erased.

Just as important, due to limits on what we can retain in our minds at one time, we drop, or lose, or forget what we were doing. And you can imagine what that does to relationships that we claim are important to us.

Finally, while multitasking, our bodies go into a bit of survival mode, and again, dump the chemicals into the blood stream. Again, our health takes the hit as the chemical soup circulates unchecked, wreaking damage to organs and systems.

E. Unmet Goals: When we sit with dreams drifting unorganized and unacheived in our minds, they trick us into thinking they are tasks unfinished. Remember that a mental image is 'real' to our minds, and as such, unmet goals act upon our minds, and our stress loads, as constant reminders of failure. Talk about stress!

We must take unmet goals out of this whirlwind of constant, subconscious pressure, and place them into a portion of our brain where they do us good rather than damage. (I discuss this in my workshop,

"Goals Set to Goals Met", and see people learn to lower their stress load, while turning their lives into what they want them to be.)

F. Debt and poverty: This portion of our mental stress load is common, subconscious, and often consciously weighty at the same time. Debt will sit in the back of our mind, dragging like a sea anchor on our joy, as well as on our ability to live well. We may fool ourselves into thinking that we have our finances under control, or that our debt is working for us, but the impact on our stress level is always negative.

G. Life Changes: Interestingly, any change in our life situation triggers the chemical release of stress response. It makes no difference to our adrenal glands if the change is positive or negative, they respond with their single minded focus on "More Cortisol! More Adrenalin!" A funeral. A vacation. A promotion. A layoff. A new child. A divorce. To the adrenal glands, change is simply change, and as such they all call for the same response.

And the more of these major life changes that occur, the more stress, and the more chemical soup, and the more damage, and the more risk for health issues as a result. In a list of risk factors published by StressMarket.com, 10 out of 43 stress factors listed were positive events. And 15 more of them were merely "changes" in the status of a life circumstance, neither positive nor negative. (See the next topic.)

What they have in common is 'change in life', resulting in stress, resulting in the cascade of effects that stress brings.

H. Life Changes: Changes in life-circumstances triggers the stress response at an emotional level. A change in housing, income level, activities, habits, diet, sleeping habits, geographical location, hobbies, and more, all trigger the same response.

I. Uncontrollable Issues: The economy, world events, weather, and other factors that impinge on our lives less personally, can trigger stress response, also. Different personality types may be more prone to experiencing these factors with more of a stress response, but they are indeed a source of stress that hits at an emotional level.

J. Internal Stress: Added to the long list of external sources of stress, is the concept of our internally generated stress. Our attitude about life can cause its own stress as we imagine the worst, stew about life, amplify negative possibilities, sweat over the what ifs, and get worked up on the inside over what may (or may not) be happening on the outside. Some of us are more prone to this than others, but what we dwell on in our minds can trigger then same cascade of stress chemicals that physical, or emotional stressors do. Remember, the mind cannot tell the difference between an imagined event and an real event.

Internal stress is what many people view as the only stress. It is what they mean when they say that they don't have any stress, or don't feel stressed. But as we have seen, internal stress if far from the only trigger that release the stress chemicals, whether we feel them or not.

There is more. Take a few minutes to Google stress factors, causes of stress, or stress ranking and you will be able to read page after page of stress factors. It is ubiquitous. Stress is everywhere. You cannot avoid stress. And because you will experience stress today, your body will experience a stress response today. And tomorrow. And next week, as well. But that's why our bodies were designed the way they are. They were designed to give us the resources we need to respond to stress, sharpening our alertness, giving a boost of strength and energy when we need it, focusing our thoughts, marshalling our resources at the areas where we need them. We just need to learn how to manage the stress response in a healthy manner. And we will discuss that in great detail in chapter 6.

Key Point #4: Stress is everywhere! You cannot escape.

But, once again, we all knew that.

Chapter 5:   How Did We Get Here?

Frustratingly, the stress issue has gotten worse in the last 100 years. Not only are we subject to more stress, but we allow ourselves less room and flexibility to deal with stress load.

My grandmother died at the age of 96. I recall talking with her about her life. I remember her saying that she came from England as a girl of 17, by herself, on a ship that steamed slowly across the Atlantic Ocean. A trip that we make in 5 hours unfolded over the course of 21 long, uncomfortable days.

And even I, at the age of 'only' 57, can remember having no television, no microwave ovens, and having to tediously dial a rotary phone, and then only when the party line was clear of the neighbors using their phone!

Look at what has changed in the last century.

We have gone from no T.V., no answering machine, no microwave, no GPS, no jet airplanes, no immunizations, no CD players or DVD players, and no computers, not to mention few antibiotics, sparse electricity, few cars, no cell phones or ipads, no McDonalds, and no overnight package deliveries, to all the extremely fast conveniences of modern life. In comparison, I just returned from Israel, where I could not only call, but email and text, and send pictures to my wife, across the globe, in seconds. Imagine life as it was for almost all of mankind's history.

When the sun went down, we went to sleep. When an emergency arose, we either made up a 'fix' for the situation, or waited days or weeks for help. When we wanted to eat, we either ate a raw fruit, or harvested, cleaned and slowly cooked the next meal. When we traveled to town, it was a major event for which we planned a whole day. To get a message to the next town would take a day, to the east coast could take a month.

Obviously, things are different now. We have an insatiable demand for "Now". We have become the "I can't wait for that" generation. Speed is everything. The epitome of the Need it Now mindset is perhaps seen in the fact that, if you don't have time to wait for one minute for your pop tart to come up from the toaster, the package recommends a microwave cooking time of 3 seconds. Three seconds!

Check out this list:

■ Communications are instantaneous, and if a person won't answer the phone, we can text, email, or leave a message in seconds.

■ Travel is nearly instantaneous. What took my grandmother several weeks, high risk, and the commitment of no return, takes us a few hours, a few bucks, and we can insure our luggage.

■ Medicine – Need a blood test? Within moments, you can have the information that used to take days. And surgeries that required hours of anesthesia and days of hospitalization, now require a local numbing, moments of microsurgery on an outpatient basis, and a half a day off from work.

■ Computers are miniaturized and so much faster. Rooms full of number crunchers are replaced by a pocket calculator. A printing job that would have taken months of man-hours can be type set, proof read, and sent to an instant, full-color printer within moments.

■ Law enforcement has seen vast changes, as well. Finger prints can be taken, analyzed, sent around the world, and compared to millions of others in data banks – in seconds. DNA still takes days to analyze, but that, too, is vastly quicker than anything found in police work in human history.

What makes this even more profound, even beyond the dramatic changes that have touched and transformed every aspect of life, is the fact that the rate of change is accelerating. Not only are we inundated with more changes, but the changes come at us at a faster and faster rate than ever before.

The rate at which computers become obsolete is a hyperbolic curve, not a simple upward slope. The rate at which we are learning new facts and information in every area of life is accelerating.

According to Industrytap.com,

> "Buckminster Fuller created the "Knowledge Doubling Curve"; he noticed that until 1900 human knowledge doubled approximately every century. By the end of World War II knowledge was doubling every 25 years. Today, nanotechnology knowledge is doubling every two years and clinical knowledge every 18 months. But on average, human knowledge is doubling every 13 months. According to IBM, the build out of the "internet of things" will lead to the doubling of knowledge every 12 hours."

This is amazing. Breathtaking, in fact. How can mankind hope to keep up with this vast expansion of knowledge? And how can we hope to keep up with the morality of how to use this expansion of knowledge? For instance, we now know how to clone, how to use fetal parts to fight diseases, how to build devastating weapons, how to map genes and change them. But the morality behind the use of this knowledge is untested, and may lead to grossly dubious uses of these tools.

And, of course, all of this leads to massive amounts of stress as we look on and watch actions take place, policies and laws are enacted, and lives are impacted by this amazing march toward god-like abilities to manipulate our physical and mental environment.

So, the world is changing. And it's changing faster and faster. And all of this change acts as an inescapable stressor on our minds and bodies. Stress call for action. It demands a response from our organs and glands – to either fight back, or run away. We are biologically programmed to respond to things that happen around us, and our neurochemistry is designed to prepare us for that action.

Another way to look at the way our body responds to stressors is to think in terms of general body responses, and actual physiological and structural changes that occur in response to our bodies.

As we have seen, the general responses that our bodies undertake, happen whether the stressor (change in our environment) is negative or positive. Whether we win the lottery or crash our car, our body releases the exact same chemicals into our blood stream. All stressors demand, and receive, the exact same response from our adrenal glands and other stress-responsive glands. And we saw an extensive list of what that does to our physiology in chapter 3. The intensity of the response may vary with the intensity of the stressor, but the chemistry is the same.

So a car crash will trigger a bigger chemical dump into our system than stubbing your toe, but trigger they will. A win of a million dollar jackpot may evoke a larger response than finding a shiny nickel on the sidewalk, but both do the job. Chemistry flows, the body responds, and presto! You are ready for a battle or a party.

The stressors of life are growing faster than we can keep up with them. They surround us. They are subtle, and they are in our faces. They are slowly eroding the resources that we keep in reserve for emergencies. And, unless we deliberately do something about it, they are winning.

There is a real battle going on here, and many of us don't even know it's happening. Stress is winning. Sumpin's Gotta Give!!

Key Point #5: Life is charging, and charging downhill.

Did we already know that?

Chapter 6: What is to be done?

Since stressors are everywhere, and stressors cause our bodies to respond in predictable ways that, due to our modern lifestyles, tend to injure our physical bodies, what are we to do?

Good news! There are actually two things we can do that will tame the stress monster.

First, we can reduce the stress load by changing some of the pieces of our lifestyle. And second, we can learn practical methods to manage the stress and stress chemicals that are in our lives.

So let's get practical. Let's dive into the first area of what we can do to get the stress issue on our team, rather than just letting it beat us up year after year. What can we do to decrease the stress load? Plenty!

But one of the challenges in lowering the actual amount of stress we have in our lives is that it requires – yup, you guessed it – change. And what is the simplest definition of stress? Again – change. So the catch is that to diminish stressors in our lives, we have to introduce yet more change, and, as we discussed in chapter one, you can't have change without stress chemicals being downloaded into your blood stream! A conundrum, if I've ever heard of one.

So we must choose carefully. What are we going to pick to change in our effort to lower stress. The big stressors in life include our job, our health, our relationships and our finances. These big four are by far the greatest sources of stress in modern life. Part of the problem is that they are either very difficult to change, or very stressful to change.

Changing your career path involves much planning, training and potential upset. Certainly there are times when a complete change in career is appropriate, but get some wise counsel on that before burning bridges that will cost you in the long run.

Changing relationships also brings with it a lot of inner turmoil, and may very well not be a wise thing to do. Far wiser to invest in improving our relationships by means that will improve the stress load without having to make massive changes in who we hang out with. Counseling, or books on wise boundaries (See "Boundaries" by Henry Townsend), or other aspects of healthy relationships may go a long way to easing that source of stress in your life. The investment in your health will pay extra dividends in lowering your stress load.

Changing your health is a viable option for only some people, though there are certainly things to do to accomplish strides in that direction. I discuss that in detail in my book "Reservoir of Better Health".

And finally, changing your finances is a challenge as well. If it were easy, we would all do it, right?

While this book cannot tackle the topic and do it any justice, a couple resources to help with financial stress might include books by David Ramsey, and a little book on alternate incomes called "The Four Year Career".

What I do want to spend some time on in this book is two "micro stressors". The irritating, nagging little stressors that we can change and improve without tipping over the stress wagon in the process. These things are stressors that seem to always be present, and yet are usually overlooked because they individually fail to capture our attention like the big four (our job, our health, our relationships and our finances) do.

Here are two categories of order that may bring some sanity to a crazy life. The topics I have labeled "Simplify" and "Organize", though those titles may be a bit misleading if you are jumping to conclusions about what they entail. Let's unpack each of them.

1) Simplify – finding that less is actually more, more peace of mind, more space, more tranquility – all from recognizing the value of simplifying our lives. To quiet our hearts and minds is to find a reservoir of peace that we can take with us through the day.

"Too much" is a disease in our culture. The tendency to pack junk into every nook and cranny of our calendars, our drawers, and our minds is a temptation, a habit, and a curse. So simplifying includes finding the places where we squirrel away useless junk and getting rid of it. Or at least putting it in order so that it is not nibbling away in the back of our minds like a chipmunk grinding away at the insulation in the attic of our brains.

So, simplifying our lives includes tackling our chaotic life, one storage spot at a time and bringing order and a little bit "less" into it. If this thought makes your palms sweat and your breathing quicken, don't panic. Start small and watch the grip of "too much" loosen and then relax from around your heart.

Start with a single drawer. Every home has a drawer where odds and ends accumulate. Things that you use often enough to keep, but rarely enough that we forget what all is in there. Go to that drawer with a small garbage bag, and a determination to set it straight. You don't need to get rid of much, but what you find in there that you have not used in three months or more should either be pitched, or placed neatly in its proper place. That place may be back in the drawer, or it may be in a better place in your home. But when you have gone through the whole drawer, it should be neater than it was, and hold less than it did before your approached it 20 minutes earlier.

Now that it's done, the drawer is neater, you can find what you need from that drawer, the drawer opens and closes easily, and if you sit down and listen to your heart, you can sense that your shoulders feel a bit lighter. You have taken your first step toward a lighter stress load.

If you really liked that project, take on another drawer. Or pick a closet. But wait another day until you pick an entire room, or your garage.

I just searched Amazon for books on organizing and got over 10,000 results. Do not order all of them. But there are certainly a lot of resources available to help you bring order to a chaotic "Too Much" life.

Now, what about our calendars? There are two components to our schedules that contribute to our stress load. One is, again, too much. In this context, too many things to do. And the second is 'owning' commitments to the wrong things.

We must learn the value, and the morality of saying "no" to both too much and to the wrong things. God did not place either you or me on this earth to do everything. He only calls us to do the few right things. The things that will fulfill us, and bring a smile to His face. Certainly, there are a lot of things – very good things – available for us to do. But we must learn to quietly listen to Him, and to our own heart, in order to choose only the right things.

I have been guilty of this many times in the past. I said yes to so many good things, that the important and great things got crowded out. I sacrificed time with my own family because I got so caught up in committees and groups that sounded to fulfilling to me. I knew I could do those things well, so I just kept saying yes, until I was a stranger in my own home. I still have to fight that tendency, so every year or so I look at my list of commitments and try to pare it down. I heard of one very successful business man who has a scheduled habit of saying no to one thing every week. And if there is no new demand on his time, he deliberately takes one thing off of his commitments. This mind set leaves room in our calendar and in our mind to think, to be and to respond to incidental stressors that pop up.

Another aspect of this anti-stress campaign in our calendars is to schedule into our daily calendar empty time. As though it were an appointment, enter a half hour of blank time into your schedule. Perhaps two 15 minute slots of empty space, one in the middle of the morning, and one at the end of each day.

All by itself, these buffer times will bring ease to your mind, and you will feel your brain unwinding a bit as you realize that you have time to do what you have on your plate.

Absolutely refuse to multi-task. To the best of your ability, focus on the one thing in front of you with 100 percent of your focus. Give your all to what you are looking at right in that moment. This gives value to the people you are talking to, and value to the task you are doing.

Break large jobs into pieces. Make each large project into tasks that can be done in one sitting, and list them in the proper order.

Finally, if you are at all able, schedule the first part of your day for working on those tasks. Tackle a couple items that can actually be finished and get them done first thing in the morning, and then move on to other, more complicated tasks. Then schedule a defined time slot during your day to answering texts and "working on" social media. This will avoid the black hole of social media. Social media has a purpose, but it can be addictive and destructive to your productivity. By scheduling in a set and limited time for it, you will keep a manageable distance between the giant time-sucking vacuum of social media and your priceless minutes.

Next, when faced with opportunities of good things to do, only say yes to the ones that are good for you. Avoid stressful commitments that rob you of peace and relaxation. There are people out there who can tackle those things and find joy in them. Just because these jobs are available, and are good, and need to be done, does not mean that you need to do them. Again, the word "no" comes in handy. Use it.

There are polite ways to say no, of course. You don't have to feel guilty about it. You can legitimately say that you need to consider it, pray over it, or get advice on it. Never feel that you need to say yes, much less that you need to say yes under pressure to decide right away.

And then you can honestly say that that opportunity, while an honor, doesn't fit into your schedule. "Thank you for considering me for that. But I don't think I can do that job justice without robbing from my other commitments."

Why, it's even okay to say something as simple and true as, "No, I don't think I can do that." You and I have the right, and even the responsibility, to say 'no' to things that you and I feel are not in our best interest. We don't have to explain it if we don't want to. We don't have to feel guilty. We simply need to know ourselves and to be true to the important things in our lives.

Does competition make you uncomfortable? Then say no. How about public speaking? Say no. How about considering your gifts and talents, and saying yes to only those things that you can honestly feel fit in that mix.

And when you do say yes, only do so if you can continue giving your critical priorities the attention they deserve, and also still protect the schedule buffers that you already fought to put in place.

Another way to lessen stress is to avoid encounters that rob your peace. These encounters may be certain people who are consistently raising topics that raise your hackles, or they may be media outlets that tighten your chest as you interact with them. News channels deliberately choose topics that are full of conflict in order to entice, and then trap, viewers.

For me, the biggest source of this aspect of stress is a combination of people and media – namely, facebook encounters with people who post items that I feel passionately about. When people I care about post items that I disagree with, I feel my peace leaving. I can literally feel my stomach tighten, my chest clench, and my blood pressure rise. I say to myself, "What? They believe that?!", and I feel that I must respond, and set them back on the right course. LOL

I have learned two things about this. One – no one has ever changed their mind as a result of a facebook discussion. And two – such discussions always result in walls built between people. It's just not effective as a debate medium. And it's destructive to relationships. I have learned (okay, I'm still learning) that it is best to just walk away.

One more facet to lessening the stress load by simplifying: talk less. I don't mean to imply that we benefit by avoiding conversations. I mean God gave us twice as many ears as mouths for a reason. I came up with this algebraic equation to mathematically prove the idea. **1M x 2E = W**, where **M** = Mouth, **E** = Ears, and we solve for **W**. (One mouth times two Ears equals Wisdom!)

I am learning to offer advice only when asked. Another way to look at this is to get more advice than you give. Whether it is on social media or face to face, people will not hear or receive, much less appreciate what they have not asked for.

Decreasing the load of stressors that we carry through the daily grind takes discipline and insight, both of which we can have. By becoming aware of our true purpose in life, and then aligning our physical surroundings, our schedules and our interactions with people with that purpose we find there is less emotional dissonance within our hearts. Our bodies no longer sense that mental friction between who we are, and what we are doing, and we stop producing the quantity of the stress hormones that was slowly killing us before.

Simplify your surroundings and your schedule, say no to the right things, and your 'yeses' will be much more effective. We can live longer and better by doing less of the wrong things and doing the right things better.

2) Organize – the second way to lower the stress load is to organize the various pieces of your life into packages of life that you can access and implement with minimal strain on your resources of time and attention.

Now that you have simplified a bit, and explored the idea that it's okay to do less and yet have a more fulfilling and productive life, what's next? Next is to learn how organizing your mind can help lower your stress load dramatically.

The term organize may take you with a groan back to the last topic of what we called simplify, but in our current context, I want to use organize to lead you toward a mind that can focus on what is really important to you. And there are basically two facets to this task of organizing your mind. The first is to find and grasp your life purpose, and the second is to focus on that purpose in every decision you make. Are you ready?

Let's dive in.

Organizing by means of knowing your life purpose: Life purpose can be defined as the reason why you are here. Why does your life matter? What makes you come alive when you envision yourself doing it? These are broad questions, and may be overwhelming to consider. But let's invest a few minutes and break them down into exercises that you can do to define your own life purpose.

Now don't tune me out. As important as knowing what your purpose is, don't feel that this is a chore that you've got to grind out like a 10th grade algebra assignment – "and show your work". <u>Susan Biali M.D.</u> puts it this way, " It's not something to be forced, or something to actively worry about "having to" find. I like to think of it as a treasure hunt, a perfectly paced adventure with your eyes and heart wide open. Be curious. Enjoy the process. Marvel at life and its richness as you go along."

First, some ground rules. Your purpose must be bigger than you are. By that, I mean that your purpose, if fulfilled, should out last your own life. This means that your purpose statement should be less material, and more spiritual. It should impact more than just your own comfort level. It should effect more people than just yourself. And, ideally, it should impact in a widening circle of influence as time passes.

Now this does not mean that your purpose disqualifies material items from your goals list, but for right now, let's think big. What drives you? What reason would God have for creating you? 50 years after your eventual demise, what would you want people to remember you for?

Here's a question that may help you find your true purpose. Ask yourself, "What do I like to do so much that I'm willing to be ridiculed for doing it?" If something is so deep in your heart that you would do it even if nobody understood or encouraged you, it is probably there because it is part of your genetic makeup. And if you are made that way, you will probably be happier if you can find a way to be involved in that, in some fashion, throughout your life.

Spend some time thinking and journaling your response to that question. And then ask yourself this series of questions:

"What do people say I'm really good at?"

"What do I enjoy doing even when I'm not getting paid for it or acknowledged for it?"

And finally, "At the end of my life, what would I regret most if I had never done it?"

As you think on these questions, and the ambulations your mind will take you on as you ponder their answers, you will find patterns. There will be things, activities, likes and dislikes, organizations, people and even attitudes that you find common among several of the question lines.

And these can reveal facets of your original blueprint.

From this time of introspection you will uncover things about yourself that can help guide you in future decisions. By knowing what you were made to do, you can focus your energies and resources on opportunities that bring you joy and fulfillment, rather than just your next paycheck.

I'm not knocking the importance of your next paycheck, but if you can begin to craft your life to fit your purpose, you can find peace and joy in the process of earning those paychecks. And a life of joy with a paycheck is far better than a paycheck without joy and fulfillment.

Try to craft a purpose statement by filling in the following sentence.

I was put here on this earth to

_____. Or:

I exist to _____. Or:

The reason I get up each morning is to

_____.

This purpose statement is not permanent. It is a work in progress, and will change as you experience more, and as you hone your understanding about what brings you joy and a sense of "Ahh. That was worth doing."

Let me share with you my own current purpose statement. But promise that you won't read it until you have spent at least a half hour working on your own. I'll put it in parentheses to make it a little harder to read accidentally:

(I am here to gently help people find truth, and to lovingly live in that truth as consistently as possible.)

Once you have a life purpose statement, you can start to build life goals that will lead you to a life that was well lived. Which leads us to the second facet of organizing your life – setting goals.

Write a draft of your life purpose statement here before going on:

Organizing by means of setting goals: There are five steps to setting goals that will change your life. I teach a workshop on this that walks you through each step, but here I will take you through the process in enough detail for you to get there on your own.

First, sit down with a blank sheet of paper and a pen. Set a timer for 5 minutes, and start writing. Write every single thing you want to accomplish in your life. Everything.

I recall when I first received that challenge, my reaction was that I would continue writing for hours, and use several pages of paper. Don't fear that. You will find that you will write fast and furious for about 90 seconds, and then you will start to slow down, then to think harder, and then to wrack your brain for a new goal. When you do slow down to a slower pace, consider these categories for new ideas.

What do you want to learn? To do? To teach?

Where do you want to go?

When do you want to retire? With how much money?

What is your dream house? Car? Vacation?

What do you want to give to charity? Who do you wish you could help? What organizations do you wish you could give to?

Do you want to be a board member of some organization?

What skill do you want to develop?

Think of goals that would involve your physical health, your career, your spiritual life, your family and relationships, and your finances.

Consider goals for the next year, 5 years, 20 years, and goals that will impact the world 50 years after you are gone.

Think big. And think small. Nothing is off the table in this phase of your goal setting. And do not judge your goals here as being valid or not, as being righteous or not, as being selfish or not, or as being achievable or not. Write – Them – ALL – Down.

This list is called your **Master Goal List**, and it is plastic. You can add to it any time. You can change is later. I don't recommend that you take items off the list, but you can always build it longer. This list is not a commitment to do everything on it. So leave them on. Don't critique it. Don't second guess it. Just write everything that comes to your mind.

So for right now, take the full five minutes and work it.

How many did you come up with? In my first go at this I came up with a list of 42 goals. They ranged from owning a Dodge Viper to going to Israel. I listed learning about coin collecting, and building a school in a remote village in South Sudan.

Okay, next is to take this list, and put the items into categories. The categories can be any five facets of your life that bring balance to your own wheel of life. I like to use:

Career / Finances – what do you want your career to look like in the rear view mirror?

Relationships – what do you want your family and friendships to look like?

Emotional / Spiritual – what do you want to accomplish that is physically intangible?

Physical – what do you want to accomplish with your physical being?

Altruistic Goals – what things do you want to do that benefit others?

Other goals might include Knowledge, Social, or Education. You get to choose the five categories, but try to see that they encompass a balanced life, not focused entirely on material or financial success.

Now take each item from your **Master Goals List** and place it into one of these categories. Look them over to see that you have something in each category, and that there is some semblance of balance between them.

Okay! That's progress!

Next you are going to look at each list and prioritize them by taking one goal from each category. This will give you a list of 5 active goals that you can work on at any given time. So look over the list of **Career / Financial** and select the one you want to work on first.

Then take one from the **Relationships** list. And so on. One way to decide which goal to choose is to compare the goal to your life purpose statement. Does it support your purpose? If so, it can go onto your 'short list', and still act in a stress lowering fashion.

It may also help to choose some quick and easy goals, and not all huge, long-term goals. This avoids some frustration in the early days of working your goals program.

Place each goal at the top of its own blank page. These five pages are your **Active Goal Worksheets**.

Take one of these goals and start to work it by doing the following:

1) Word the goal so that it is very specific. So don't say, "I am going to retire." Say, "I am retiring at age 61, with $500,000 in the bank."

2) Word it in present tense. This triggers the mind to find ways to make this sentence true in fact. So don't say, "I will travel to Rome." Say "I am traveling to Rome."

3) Word it in a positive, so that the sentence is triggering positive energy rather than negative. So rather than, "I won't smoke anymore," say, "I am comfortably tobacco free."

4) Word it so that it is measurable. You have to know when the goal is accomplished. So don't say, "I want to lose weight." Say, "I am losing 15 pounds."

Next, on each **Active Goal Worksheet**, fill in the following information. Each piece of this information has an impact on your subconscious. They all add up to a deeper agreement that you will get this done. They are ways to fire up your brain (See the paragraph on the Reticular Activating System, below) and put it to work, drawing into your life the energy and other resources to get your goals done.

They are like lighting the fuse on the powder that will drive your goals.

1) **Due By Date** – put a date by which you will accomplish this goal.

2) **Accountability** – who can you talk with periodically who will remind you how important your goals are.

3) **Describe** the goal in as much detail as you can. Incorporate how it will look when it is accomplished. How it will sound, feel, even smell. How will it feel to your heart when it is done? Find a picture of the goal if that is practical, and attach it to its **Active Goal Worksheet**.

4) And then break the goal down into **steps**. Each step should be a distinct task that can be done in one sitting. Some goals will only have one or two steps, others will have several, or many steps. Put them in order

so that you can tell at a glance what step you will need to work on next.

There is an area of your brain that is responsible for your focus and attention. It is the inputfilter that is responsible for letting certain information through to your consciousness, and sending other input and data down to subconscious. This collection of brain cells and connections is situated at the core of the brain stem and is called the **Reticular Activating System (RAS).**

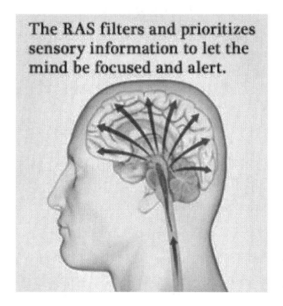

The RAS filters and prioritizes sensory information to let the mind be focused and alert.

The RAS is the part of the brain that is the center of awareness and motivation. (Interestingly, general anesthetics work by tightening the filter of the RAS.) The activity of this system is crucial for maintaining the state of consciousness. It is crucially involved with conscious experience. The RAS is the neurologic reason why you start to see more cars of the same model as the one you just bought. That car model is now tagged by your brain to let it through the filters.

Those cars were there all the time, even before you bought yours, but your RAS filtered them out into the information din that holds data unimportant to you.

This filter system is imperative to avoid being overwhelmed by the sheer volume of information collected by your eyes, ears, thoughts, and other senses. In fact, some mental illnesses are thought to be caused or compounded by a breakdown of the filter. Masses of too many sounds and sights get past the filters and overwhelm the brain.

We can train our RAS to be more lenient toward certain information. Setting goals is one way to let the RAS know that you want to allow in all of the data and information that pertains to moving toward your goals. Thus, you become more aware of opportunities and paths that move you in that desired direction.

Our system of goal setting is one way to prime the RAS filter to pass chosen information through the filters that will help you achieve your goals.

Now, with this understanding of how you can make your brain, specifically the Reticular Activating System, work for you and your goals, let's finish up the goal setting process.

From the list of task-sized steps, select one "**Next Step**" from each **Active Goal Worksheet**. Write each of those five next steps on your to-do list. If you have a daily to-do list put them on for today.

There is a distinct pleasure in checking off a task on a to-do list. And even more so as you watch the list of steps on each **Active Goal Worksheet** fall before the onslaught of your gradual, relentless pressure.

Slowly, surely, and with great satisfaction you will see your goals take form in manifest reality, one day at a time.

By having a **Life Purpose Statement** that brings focus and consistency to your life journey, and by setting goals that put effective action into your daily routine, you have lowered your stress load considerably. You are now in the driver's seat of your life, rather than letting chance and outside forces move you in random directions.

Key point #6: Less stress means better health.

But, then, we already knew that!

Chapter 7: How to manage stress

Marlene had stress enough for any dozen normal people. It told in her health. She struggled with her blood pressure, her cholesterol, her weight, her energy level and more. She finally decided to change some things. She dropped most of the inflammatory foods from her diet, she started moderate exercise on a regular basis, she lost 37 pounds, and she began journaling. Within two months, her health, her energy and her blood chemistry numbers all came back down to within normal limits. She will attest – there is something that you can do about stress, and it does have direct impact on your health.

There are some things that we can do to lower the stress load. Even without making large changes in our life circumstances, there are at least two practical ways to help our body stop pumping out so many stress chemicals. We discussed the value of establishing a life purpose statement, and of setting goals in the last chapter.

But even with the most clear of purpose statements, and even with steady progress on your goals lists, there is still 'stuff' in your life that will trigger the adrenal glands. Remember, any change, and any challenging situation will result in more stress response, and a more toxic chemical soup of stress.

So we still have a potential problem. Those chemicals can be useful, but if they just swish around and around in your arteries and veins, they will cause trouble. They will affect your health in a negative way.

Thankfully, there are specific and practical things you can do to lower the concentration of those chemicals and the impact that they have on your health. As we discuss the list, watch for three of them that you can consciously incorporate into your daily routine. Pick three that appeal to you. Choose a total of three that will be enjoyable, that you can actually look forward to doing. If you pick one that is a chore, you are much less likely to continue doing it. You can occasionally swap them around for variety, but get three of these into your routine, and make them a habit starting today.

■ **Sweat it out - Exercise:** So good for us in so many ways, yet, we are often haphazard about doing it. There are actually 5 different exercise components to work on, including:

> ■ **Cardio** – aim for 150 minutes weekly of heart-rate-increasing activity

> ■ **Resistance** – free weights, machines or elastic bands

> ■ **Spinal stabilization** – keep your spine healthy with exercises. Get my videos on this at www.ChangeYourWorld.us

> ■ **Core stability** – I recommend plank exercises. Again go to my web site, and click on the link to my videos

■ **Balance re-training** – crucial for aging and preventing falls. But start now. Don't wait until you notice your balance failing.

Get some information on each of them in order to do them effectively and safely. I discuss each of them in more detail in my book "Reservoir of Better Health".

■ **Write it up:** Keeping a journal in which to share your private soul in a safe place helps get stress-inducing thoughts out of your head and onto paper where they are less threatening and less damaging. Invest 20 minutes, three times weekly, to journal, and drop the levels of stress toxins. If it seems overwhelming, or you come up blank on what to write, consider answering questions such as:

■ What went well today? What went badly?

■ Specifically, how can I do it better the next time?

- Who blessed my life today? Who did I bless?

- What event stands out in my mind? What did I think about that event? What did I feel about it?

- What was the high point of the day? The low point?

■ **Sleep on it - Rest right:** It usually takes about 7-8 hours to get the 4 or 5 complete sleep cycles that are necessary for adequate sleep. Dark, quiet, good posture – these are some components of good sleep. This is necessary for healing and regeneration of stressed tissues and organs. Refer to that chapter in "Reservoir of Better Health" for more information on good rest.

■ **Naps:** Power down, visualize a favorite positive memory, and relax specific muscles for five minutes at some point in the day. These short breaks renew us far beyond the small time investment would seem to.

■ **Talk it out - Express:** This is much like journaling in that it gets stressful thoughts out of our head. Find a person who you can trust to keep it to themselves, and talk it over. But be careful not to use this as an excuse to become a chronic whiner.

■ **Neural Integrity:** The nerve system is one of the two major pathways by which we deal with stress. Misalignments in the spine impact this information super-highway. Get your spine checked and tuned up at least once a month.

■ **Think right:** It has been said that our thoughts are like birds. You can't keep them from flying by, but you can keep them from building a nest in your hair. You have the authority to choose what you rent your head space to. You have the power and the responsibility to reject harmful, negative thoughts, and replace them with healthy, positive ones. This is where having a list of affirmations or verses to think on comes in handy. (See Appendix A for a list of suggested affirmations.)

■ **Speak right:** In the same way, use positive words when you comment on yourself and on those you care about. We can get in a habit of saying derogatory comments, such as "I'm so bad at directions." Or, "I never could hit a golf ball." Stop that! Speak positive truth over yourself and your people. Words matter. Use good ones to describe yourself.

■ **Rub it out - Massage:** There is something about human touch that lowers stress levels. Treat yourself to a half hour massage once in a while. And in between, a worthy goal is to get/give away 10 hugs each day. Hugs are much like a recharge for the soul, and they do a ton for lowering stress.

■ **Spiritual Health:** An integral part of holistic health is to take care of the body, heart and spirit. They work together like the strands of a web. You must not ignore any of the three, or imbalances begin to force a wobble into our lives. Take the time to keep your spirit healthy with time spent quietly with God, with holy scripture, with verses.

■ **Pets:** Of course, it depends on the pet. But having an animal who loves you, who you can care for, and by whom you can be cared about, is a definite stress reducer. A dog I lived with once, was an exception. Her tendency to snap at me in thanks for the food I set down for her each morning, her practice of climbing over a five foot chain link fence, and to wander terrorizing the neighbors, earning a death threat from one of them – did nothing to lessen my stressin', let me tell you. Choose wisely. Perhaps a gold fish?

■ **Eat right:** The edible stuff we stuff into our mouths can either detoxify or poison us. Choose live foods, good-quality supplements, and plenty of pure water hydration every day. You don't have to live the life of a vegetarian, but shift your choices toward fruits and vegetables, decreasing processed sugars and carbs. This will, in turn, shift your body chemistry toward less inflammation, less acidity, and less stress.

■**Essential Oils:** This topic is exploding in popularity right now. And rightfully so! With the national trends toward less effective medications, toxicity in our environment, and the growth of super bug bacteria and viruses, this natural and effective way to bring health back to our lives is timely and important.

To learn more on this topic, visit www.YoungLiving.com

This company produces the high quality oils that get great results, and has a ton of information to help you get up to speed. (If you join, I'd love you to use us as your referring member. Use 2784644 as our membership number.)

So – there is a list of practical ways to lower stress chemistry in your life. Sometimes, however, the stress has accumulated to the point where you need more than that. What follows are more advanced steps to interrupt an out-of-control, stressed out life. These ideas work, but are more involved, so get someone to coach you through these if you decide to work them into your life. A holistic Chiropractor, a Naturopath, or a Nutritional counselor may be options to explore.

■ **Detox** – a detox regimen can be a simple 3 day fast, a flush using teas or water, or a 30 day reboot. For more guidance with these contact us at DrRoost@yahoo.com

■ Find and eliminate the allergens – an **elimination diet** eliminates possible allergens, one at a time, for a period of a week. During that week take NONE of that food type in, and drink plenty of water to flush. Typical toxins might be sugar, milk, gluten, soy or wheat.

■ Clean out the **filters** – Our bodies have filter systems that are responsible for cleaning out our internal environment. These include kidneys, liver, lungs and skin, and can get overloaded or "clogged up". Cleaning them out on a regular basis is important, and can be done with a regimen similar to detox. Again, get some help to implement this.

■ Kale, Green tea, Gabba, Adrenal extract, CoQ10 and others – these **supplements** are helpful with resetting and rebooting our metabolism and inner, chemical health.

Key Thought #7: There are specific, practical ways to deal with the chemical soup.

Did you know that?

Chapter 8: Benefits to lowering stress

As we saw with Marlene, there are definite benefits to lowering the stress load and managing the stress chemistry. Here are some further, specific outcomes that might motivate us to manage our stress better. (TheMentalFitnessCenter.com website was a good resource for this section.)

1. **Weight Loss.** We have seen (Chapter 2) that stress is a strange monster. An example of this is the fact that stress can cause either weight gain or weight loss. It does this by messing with our hormones, our energy level, metabolic rate, appetite, and thyroid function.

2. **Joy of Life.** This one may seem obvious, but it's too important to leave out. Stress robs us of our health and energy, and thus our joy. At

times it happens so slowly that we don't notice it until we either compare it to how we were years ago, or until we suddenly get rid of it. At that point we say, "Ahhh. So that's how life can be."

3. **Cancer Protection.** Stress impacts our immune system and can be implicated in compromising ability to fight off everything from colds to cancer. The sooner we get it under control, the sooner our immune system can get back on the job, protecting us from monsters we want no part of.

4. **Sleep the Good Sleep.** People under a great deal of stress often have interrupted sleep patterns. We know what a blessing good quality sleep is. Getting stress under control is one step toward getting back to sweet dreams.

5. **Life Expectancy.** A study from the University of Florida puts it this way: **Heart disease patients with lower mental stress are less likely to experience a decrease in blood flow to the heart, which can increase the risk of**

dying three-fold. Added to the improvement in our immune function, and we can see that stress management literally saves lives.

6. **Better Relationships.** This is an area that most stress victims are in strong denial over. The majority will tell you, "My relationships don't suffer any because of my stress They'll even say, "I keep it hidden from everyone else – no one knows the stress I'm under." However, that's like hiding a gorilla in a carton of eggs. It always leaves a mess, and it's almost as miserable for those in the vicinity of the over-stressed person as it is for the stressed person who is stomping around, breaking eggs.

7. **A healthier heart.** The Institute of HeartMath in Boulder, CO. found that "hypertensive workers who participated in a 16-hour stress reduction program experienced a significant drop in blood pressure." Furthermore, they benefited from a more positive outlook and a greater sense of peacefulness.

Positive outlook + Greater sense of peacefulness + Healthier heart = Better life. A no-brainer!

8. **Relief from aches and pains.** According to EveryDayHealth.com, "Stress and pain are often closely linked. Each one can have an impact on the other, creating a vicious cycle that sets the stage for chronic pain and chronic stress. So, part of getting pain relief is learning how to better manage stress. Lots of studies support the conclusion that what happens in the brain – depression, anxiety, being stressed out – can increase pain."

In the same way, lowering our stress load, makes a positive impact in objective pain levels.

9. **Increased Memory.** Want to remember names and dates better? Want to perform better at work? Deal with your stress! There are many research outcomes that show that those with lower stress levels perform better on tests than those who are carrying tons of stress.

10. **A Better Outlook.** When a person suffers from stress they don't look forward to birthdays, holidays, their favorite team in the playoffs, or their old fun hobbies – nothing excites them.

Key thought #8: There are real and practical benefits to lowering our stress level.

Of course, we knew that!

Chapter 9: Finding a Balance

We began this book with a comment on the dual nature of stress. It is our friend. And it is our enemy. It helps us, and it harms us. Stress prepares us for challenges, and it degrades our health in significant ways.

So how do we live with this paradox of living with stress? How do we live our lives, encounter the stressors, take the benefits and avoid the traps? The answer lies in living in a balance between avoiding stress entirely, and being buried under the load of damaging chemistry that results from stress out of control.

First, we can find a balance of the amount of stress in our lives.

Balancing for an ideal stress load: Just as with muscles, there is a balance between too much stress and too little. With too much, we start to tear and rupture and break down muscle fibers. With too little, we begin to atrophy and lose muscle mass and muscle strength. Finding the sweet spot of just the right amount of work to keep our muscles toned and strong and supple is an important part of our physical health regimen.

In exactly the same way, there is an ideal amount of stress to keep our bodies exposed to. Too much and we start to experience the issues we discussed in chapter 3. Too little, and again, negative things begin to happen. We lose the ability to function at our peak potential without a bit of exposure to those same chemicals that cause damage if out of balance.

According to lessstress.net, just as we saw in Chapter One, there is a level of stress that maximizes our ability to perform most of the tasks we face.

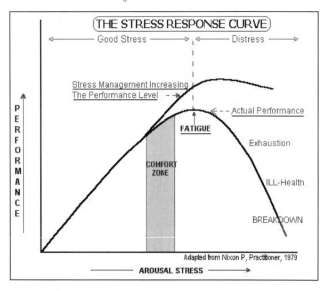

THE STRESS RESPONSE CURVE

← Good Stress → ← Distress →

Stress Management Increasing
The Performance Level →

← - - Actual Performance

P
E
R
F
O
R
M
A
N
C
E

FATIGUE

Exhaustion

COMFORT
ZONE

ILL-Health

BREAKDOWN

Adapted from Nixon P, Practitioner, 1979

← AROUSAL STRESS →

With just the right amount of stress we get the pre-game jitters. We get just a little bit nervous before a big presentation. We get just a little edgy when we know that we must perform our best – and that's a good thing. The chemical soup is dribbling into our blood in an optimal mixture, bringing a sharpness to our thinking, oxygen to our muscles, and keeping non-critical functions damped down so that we don't waste resources that we can better use in the task at hand.

Finding the right amount of stress to live with is challenging. And even when we can consciously find where that 'sweet spot' is, can we deliberately and consistently monitor and maintain that balance? It takes introspection, awareness of our life purpose, and a finely developed skill at saying "no" at the right moments to achieve it. But with practice and perhaps some advice from trusted advisors and friends, it can be done.

Second, we can learn tools to manage the stress chemicals that are being released. In Chapter Seven we listed a bunch of those tools. Choose your three, and get them into your regular routine.

Key thought #9: There is actually a "sweet spot" of stress level that allows us maximum effectiveness in life.

Did you know that?

Chapter 10: Conclusion

Let's review some of the keys that we covered in the last 100 pages.

■ Stress is everywhere, and it is far more than simply "feeling tense".

■ Too much acute stress, or prolonged, low-level, chronic stress burn us out, damage our bodies, and impact our lives in costly ways.

■ But there is a balance of stress that is important to find and maintain.

■ It saps our energy, costs money, drains productivity, and causes many diseases.

This is why we are here today, reading this manual of stress management. We aim to:

● Decrease the stress load

● Manage what's left of the Chemical soup

● Increase energy and productivity

But we must **CHANGE SOMETHING**! Simply knowing the information does us no good. In fact, the knowledge may have raised your stress level. So what are you going to do? Let me encourage you to get practical. Schedule yourself some time to:

- Set a time for evaluation and goals
- Write your goals out
- Write Next Steps to accomplish them
- Eliminate something from your life that is causing you stress
- Organize one area of your life

What are YOU going to change?

Today.

You.

When?

What are you going to change?

Do you intend to continue doing the same thing and expect a different outcome?
Keep heading the same direction and you'll surely end up with more of what you are now getting.

www.ChangeYourWorld.us has a list of links that can help you find a better balance. Go there and explore. Use some of the tools there, and you can indeed, change your world for the better.

There is work to do. But it is effective work. There is hope, for I have found in my own life that "Small changes – done consistently will result in life-changing improvements in your life."

we can and will become more than we now imagine possible!

Live Longer and Healthier

Appendix A: Affirmations

1) God has equipped me to overcome this situation.

2) I can have, and lovingly enforce, proper personal boundaries on my time and other resources.

3) It's okay, and healthy, to have down time, and to schedule quiet moments into my day.

4) I am accepted for a number of reasons:
   - I showed up.
   - I tried.
   - I gave it my best shot, with what I had to work with, in that moment.
   - I got back up.
   - I tried again.
   - I cared about someone else.

5) God made me, loves me, and wants to associate with me.

6) God is making me better every day.

7) I am valuable to God and to others (name them).

8) Better Days Ahead.

9) This, too, will pass. Facts always change. The Truth (God's promises) always stays the same.

10) I love myself, and that's okay!

11) I can say "no", and still be a loving person.

12) I am loved by God, and by _____

13) I can disagree with people and still love them, and be loved by them.

14) It is healthy to do one thing at a time, and to take the time to do it right.

15) It is okay to do a less-than-perfect job at times.

16) I am worthy of love and belonging and acceptance.

17) I can risk vulnerability, even rejection, and be okay.

Now write a few more of your own affirmations:

18)

19)

20)

21)

22)

23)

24)

Made in the USA
Charleston, SC
29 October 2015